MIND
OVER
WEIGHT

MIND
OVER
WEIGHT

THE MIRACULOUS, NEW, EASY
WAY TO LOSE WEIGHT

Martyn Dawes

metro

Published by Metro Publishing Ltd, 3 Bramber Court, 2 Bramber Road, London W14 9PB, England

First published in paperback in 2002

ISBN 1 84358 000 4

British Library Cataloguing-in-Publication Data: A catalogue record for this book is available from the British Library.

Design by ENVY

Printed in Great Britain by Clays Ltd, St Ives plc.

1 3 5 7 9 10 8 6 4 2

Papers used by Metro Publishing Ltd are natural, recyclable products made from wood grown in sustainable forests. The manufacturing processes conform to the environmental regulations of the country of origin.

ACKNOWLEDGEMENTS

I would like to thank the many friends and family who have helped me make this book possible by offering their encouragement and support, especially Sharon, my wife, and Elliot my son for putting up with me sitting at the computer for so long, 'Dad, can I have a go on the computer now!' was a common cry.

A big thank you to Chrissie Hardisty for helping me get the idea off of the ground with her constant encouragement, and technical expertise and Dr Tam Llewellyn-Edwards for use of his book *Heal Yourself and Others with Meridian Therapies*.

Lastly, but by no means least, Gary Craig who, in

developing EFT, brought a technique that will help make the world a better, brighter, and more positive place to be.

CONTENTS

• •

Foreword   11

About the Author   15

About the Book   17

Introduction   21

Diets and False Promises   23

A Brief History of Meridian Therapies   27

The Meridians

Central Meridian   34

Governing Meridian   36

Bladder Meridian   38

Gall Bladder Meridian   40

Stomach Meridian   42

Kidney Meridian **44**

Spleen Meridian **46**

Lung Meridian **48**

Large Intestine Meridian **50**

Circulation Sex Meridian **52**

Heart Meridian **54**

Small Intestine Meridian **56**

Triple Warmer or Triple Heater Meridian **58**

Unit 1

How Do I Feel Today? **61**

Unit 2

Discovering Your Truths **67**

Unit 3

Emotional Barriers **77**

Unit 4

Cravings **85**

Unit 5

Self-image **91**

Unit 6

How Is It Done? **99**

The Setup **105**

The Sequence **109**

The Gamut Procedure **123**

The Sequence Repeated **125**

Unit 7
Breathing Exercises   127
Collarbone Breathing   129
Balanced Breathing   131
Diaphragmatic Breathing   132

Unit 8
Clearing the Blocks to Weight Loss   137

Unit 9
Clearing Cravings   143

Unit 10
Clearing Emotional Barriers   149

Unit 11
Finding Personal Happiness   157

Unit 12
Your Self-image   163

Unit 13
Measuring the Change   171

Unit 14
Over to You   177

The Meridians, Points and How They Affect You   180
Troubleshooting   185
Useful Contacts and Further Information   189
Courses from LiveLifeFree   191
Other publications by the author   192

FOREWORD

● ●

EFT is a universal healing aid developed by Gary Craig in the United States from Dr Roger Callahan's Thought Field Therapy. It has its roots in applied kinesiology, a technique that links the body's main organs, their associated meridians and muscle strength. It also draws on the theories and techniques used in acupuncture and acupressure. The theory behind EFT is that the body's energy system can be corrected by realigning the meridians, the pathways in the body which carry electrical energy. You will find a detailed explanation of the different meridians later in the book.

This is nothing new — acupuncture with the use of

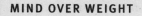
needles has been practised in the Far East for thousands of years. EFT is a psychological version of acupuncture without the needles. Instead, the body's energy system is balanced by tapping with fingertips on selected points along the energy meridians.

The most remarkable aspect of EFT for many users is the fact that it is designed so that, once learned, this simple technique can be easily done at any time, in any place, in any situation.

Martyn has broken new ground by using EFT in this book in a very innovative way. All books should inform and/or instruct and this does both. It is extremely well laid out and, when followed through, will lead the reader on a journey, discovering how the subconscious mind can affect weight, what blocks or barriers there may be and how to overcome them. Try it! What have you got to lose?

Chrissie Hardisty
Director and Trainer, Association for Meridian Therapies

The Association for Meridian Therapies (AMT) was established in 1998 to provide a register of qualified and insured practitioners throughout the UK and an insight and training in EFT together with many other Meridian Therapies.
For more information, email **chrissie@meridiantherapies.com** or visit our website: **www.meridiantherapies.org.uk**

Relax, you are *not* going on a diet.
Nobody is going to tell you what to eat,
when to eat it, and how to eat it.
You will not be told when to weigh yourself.
You will not be treated as an idiot.

You will be encouraged to take control of
your body and mind.
You will be empowered to do so.
You will be set free from your barriers to weight loss.
You will be embarking on an emotional journey.
You may laugh.
You may cry.
You will become a happier, more relaxed
and balanced person.
You will make choices.
You will become more accepting of your
body and mind.

If any of this scares you ...
well, it scares me, too!

ABOUT THE AUTHOR

· ·

I am not a doctor, dietician or counsellor.

I am a Meridian Therapist and do not consider myself
to be an expert on weight loss.

I do not believe diets work. This book shows you an
alternative way to achieve weight loss. As with most
things, you must be prepared to do the exercises
honestly.

I would advise anybody about to undergo any degree
of weight loss, including these exercises, to consult
their doctor before doing so.

Martyn J Dawes

ABOUT THE BOOK

• •

This book is set out in modules for you to work through, carefully but simply, one stage at a time. The timescale is down to you. You may be one of those people who can complete all the exercises and achieve success in a short space of time, or, like me, somebody who will read a little, do the exercise and then perhaps think on it for a few days. Best practice is to do the exercises with sincerity and honesty, totally eradicating the blocks and barriers one by one.

Wherever you see this pen symbol ✏ you can respond to prompts by writing in the book in the space provided.

The first five units are all designed to help you discover the blocks and barriers to your weight loss. These units will contain some of your hopes, desires, secrets and thoughts. **It is important that, if you do not want anybody to read them, then you should think of a good, safe hiding place for this book. Think of it now before you begin.**

Unit 6 will show you how to do the technique, whilst Units 7 to 13 are aimed at eliminating the blocks and barriers that you have identified in the earlier exercises. You may believe that some of the units will not apply to you. However, to receive the full benefit I would suggest that you attempt all of the units, even if you do not believe that they are necessary at this stage.

If you have access to the Internet, I have a weightloss workgroup at:
http://groups.yahoo.com/group/weightlossworkbook
Here you will be able to leave messages and gain advice and support from others working through the book. This group is overseen by me and I am a regular contributor, as are other Meridian Therapists. There is also a chat room, and we will be having regular get-togethers to chat and discuss any issues that you may have.

This programme *will* work if you do the techniques correctly, and are open and honest with yourself. Good luck, and best wishes for a new you!

Martyn

INTRODUCTION

●●●●●●●●●●●●●●●●●●●●●●●●●●●●●●●●●●●●●●

You are about to undergo a journey of discovery. During the course of this book, you will learn how your unconscious mind can affect your weight, why you weigh what you do, and what blocks or barriers you may have to weight loss. For many people, diets simply do not work, especially if you fall into one or more of the following categories:

☐ You can never seem to lose weight
☑ You find those last few pounds hard to shift
☑ You comfort eat

☐ You can lose weight fairly easily but put it all back on again

☑ You can never stick to a diet

☐ You eat a lot of a certain type of food (i.e. chocolate) — but this should not be confused with comfort eating

Which of these are you? Please tick those that apply to you.

Well done. You have just made the first step!

DIETS AND FALSE PROMISES

● ●

So why don't diets work for 199 out of 200 people?

• The focus is constantly on food. You are trying to lose weight and probably all you can think about is food — when can you next have a chocolate bar, or slice of your favourite cheese? How many calories in a small slice of cream cake? Can you save up enough calories/sins/ points to have a nice meal out?

• Diets also slow the metabolism. When you diet, your body thinks that food may be scarce, and processes food more slowly, whilst building up fat reserves.

• The problem is often at an unconscious level. If you are comfort eating, what are you comforting? Diets only treat the symptoms, not the cause. Why do you eat when your body does not need food?

• You may have unique blocks or barriers deep in the recesses of your unconscious mind that prevent you from losing weight.

• Diets don't deal with emotional issues. Weight gain can be triggered by a single incident, such as rejection, or other significant traumas.

• Diets don't help with confidence. You go along to your weight loss class one evening to get weighed along with countless others. You line up to discover if, that week, you are to be a success or failure; there is no middle ground. They sell you glossy magazines that contain pictures and stories of others who have lost weight using their approved methods, challenging you at an unconscious level to achieve the same success. This all costs your weekly subscription, plus a registration fee, plus buying the special frozen meals/drinks/groceries. *Undoubtedly, many people lose weight this way and I congratulate them for it.* Unfortunately, many put it all back on. If you do not know why you have failed in the past, then it is likely that you will fail again.

• Self-image is often incompatible with the weight loss you want to achieve. How you see yourself is often out of context with what you want to achieve. Can you picture yourself slim and happy, honestly? What would you look like? To start working towards this goal (if you so desire it) you would first need to picture yourself in that role, and gain acceptance in your mind that you REALLY can achieve this. This is not as difficult as you may think.

• You probably eat too much. Your stomach is only the size of a large orange. You need to become more tuned into your body and the requirements it has. Your body will tell you when to eat, how much to eat and when to stop.

A BRIEF HISTORY OF MERIDIAN THERAPIES

· ·

Meridian Therapies are by no means an original concept. A cadaver approximately 5,000 years old was recently excavated from a glacier and was found to have tattoos marking specific acupuncture points. These points have also been discovered on drawings found in caves inhabited by early man. This comes as no surprise to Meridian Therapists today, as the classic book on acupuncture is 4,500 years old. What is surprising, I suppose, is that western physicians are only just beginning to appreciate the benefits of acupuncture, when it is clearly one of the oldest forms of medicine. Meridian Therapies cover a wide range of treatments that focus on the meridian system, a sort of channelling system for the body's energies. These include acupuncture, acupressure and a whole host of new energy therapies.

1964 saw one of the developmental jumps from acupressure to these new energy therapies when George Goodheart, a chiropractor, began to investigate links between the organs of the body, meridians and muscle strength. His research led to him developing Applied Kinesiology.

In 1979, Roger Callahan used techniques based on Applied Kinesiology on a patient named 'Mary', a water phobic, whose phobia was so severe she could not go out when it rained. The result was dramatic and instant. Mary lost her water phobia instantly! She later went for a paddle in the sea.

Roger Callahan developed this further and introduced Thought Field Therapy (TFT). This involved using individually designed sequences, or 'algorithms', of tapping on particular spots. The process required a great deal of training, skill and knowledge.

In 1995, a Stanford engineer and student of Roger Callahan's technique, Gary Craig, simplified TFT into a universally applicable protocol that he calls Emotional Freedom Technique, or EFT. This technique involved just one universal algorithm sandwiched by processes known as 'The Setup' and 'The Gamut Procedure'. Applying this simple procedure, whilst focusing on the problem at hand, has proved over and over again that it is simple, concise and yet highly effective.

I first came across EFT whilst looking for alternative methods to alleviate pain. Somebody told me to try EFT, and that I could download the manual from Gary Craig's website. (See the **Contacts and Information** section at the back of this book.) I read the manual with a healthy degree of scepticism that what was in it could change lives for the better. The claim was that, by dealing with negative emotions, long-lasting and effective change could be delivered quickly. I decided to try it, and my father was to be the guinea pig! I asked him to think of an event that he wished had never happened. He replied that being made redundant 15 years earlier still left him feeling bitter. I asked him to score that bitterness on a scale of 0 to 10 and he told me that it was a 9. After 15 years, I thought that was very high, but we all carry these sorts of thoughts around with us, every day. I guarantee that if I asked you to think of an event that still carries an emotional 'hook' for you, you could think of something that scores at least above a 7, and time, the great healer, does not always do its stuff. Sometimes it just sinks deeper into our unconscious and lurks there, waiting for the opportunity to rear its head again.

I told my father that I wanted to try out this new technique and reluctantly he agreed ... and reluctantly I began. I say I began reluctantly because the process seemed weird, and if it did not work I would look stupid. We did one 'round' of the EFT sandwich and the score dropped to 6; then another round dropped the score to 4 and finally 0. I was astounded, and my father was astonished that the bitterness that he had carried for so long had gone.

I rang back a day later and it was still gone, and it has not returned since. I decided there and then that this was the thing for me and wanted to learn more. The next logical step was to become a qualified practitioner, which I achieved through one of the courses run by the Association of Meridian Therapists UK. (See the *Contacts and Information* section at the back of this book.)

I emailed a colleague who told me that when he went

to become a practitioner, he was used in front of the class as a volunteer and had burst into tears, such was the intensity of the emotion. And all of this on the first day! Hah, I thought, that would never happen to me. Well, I didn't make it to lunchtime on the first day. In a powerful example of how negative emotions can linger in the unconscious and present themselves unexpectedly, I was reduced to an absolute blubbering wreck within the first few hours! I wish to emphasise here that I am a 36-year-old man who does not cry, ever. I cannot remember ever crying, it is something I had always believed that 'real' men don't do. I was shocked, but the lesson has never been forgotten. In my private practice, I often hear clients say things like, 'I can't believe that I am telling you this,' and clients who laugh at how ridiculous the whole process seems will weep openly less than 30 seconds later when we really 'hit the point'.

EFT is an immensely powerful technique that should not be taken lightly. I give warnings in the book that must be heeded. After doing the technique for the first time, give yourself a day or two to allow your body to settle down.

I have provided a chart entitled **The Meridians, Points** *and How They Affect You,* which you will find at the back of this book. The chart will enable you to determine the direct effect that each meridian and its corresponding point will have on you physically and psychologically.

If you wish to meet a practitioner in your area, you can email me at **livelifefree@hotmail.com** or call free on 0800 083 0796 to be referred to someone suitable. This is normally an answerphone service.

The Meridians

There are 12 meridians that run in pairs mirroring each other on each side of the body. In addition, there are two further meridians that flow individually.

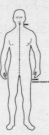
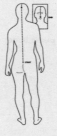
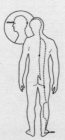
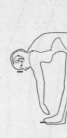
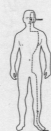
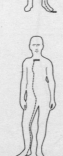
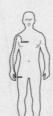
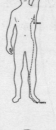
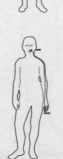
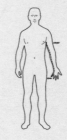
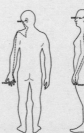
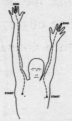

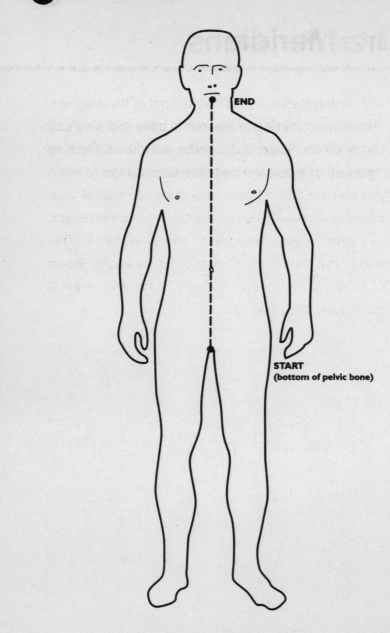

END

START
(bottom of pelvic bone)

Central Meridian

• •

The Central Meridian runs up the front of the body in a straight line starting at the pubic bone and finishing just under the lower lip. Together with the Governing Meridian, a complete loop of the body is formed when you touch the tip of your tongue on the roof of your mouth. It is also known as the Conception Vessel and can store a large amount of energy within it. This energy can then flow into the other meridians. When blocked, it can store up past traumatic events, particularly birth trauma.

Governing Meridian

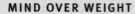

The Governing Meridian runs from the very base of the spine up the back and over the head in a straight line, coming down between the eyes and finishing just above the top lip. Together with the Central Meridian above, it forms a complete loop of the body. It is also known as a Vessel and can store large amounts of energy. Blockage may cause introvertedness and can lead to problems communicating with others. When people are stuck for something to say, they will sometimes rub the spot above the top lip inadvertently.

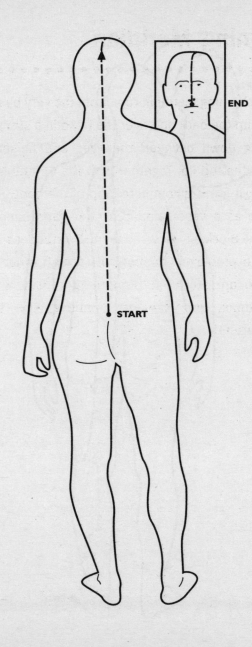

START

END

START

END

Bladder Meridian

• •

The Bladder Meridian runs from the eyebrow, up over the head and down the middle of the back. From the lower spine it flows down the back of the leg to the heel, and then along the outside of the foot ending at the little toe. It is linked with fear and courage, and also forgetfulness and impatience.

Gall Bladder Meridian

● ●

The Gall Bladder Meridian is difficult to trace, as it flows in a zigzag fashion starting at the corner of the eye and flowing down the side of the body to the fourth toe. A blockage can deplete energy but when tapped may increase determination. It aids clarity of thought but is linked with ailments such as gallstones, headaches and stiff muscles and joints.

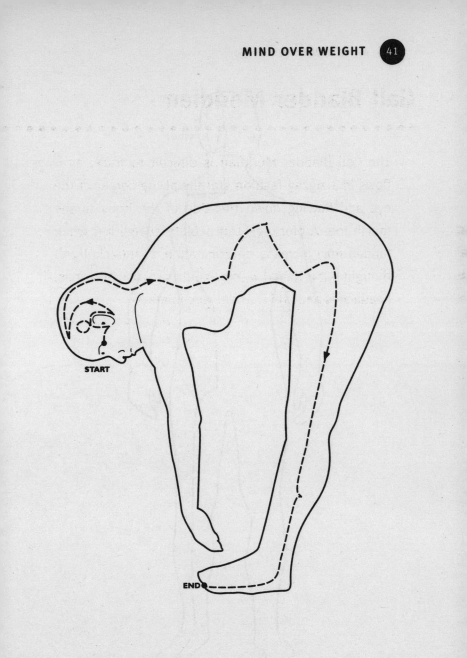

START

END

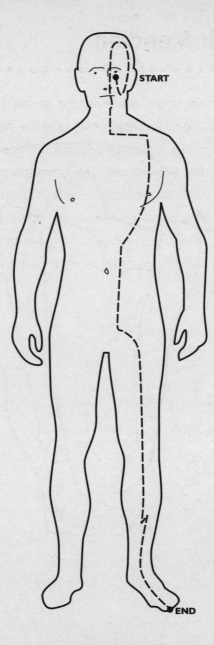

START

END

Stomach Meridian

Starting from under the eye, the stomach meridian runs along the collarbone, down over the nipple to the groin. From here it flows down the outside of the leg ending at the second toe. The stomach meridian is associated with indecisiveness, intuition and dogmatic thinking. As would be expected of this meridian, it can be linked with appetite disorders, indigestion, weight problems and vomiting.

Kidney Meridian

● ●

Poor decision-making, lack of willpower and a whole host of physical symptoms relate to this meridian. I find that my clients tend to like the collarbone point being tapped, and it is this meridian that flows at the collarbone point. Starting under the foot, the Kidney Meridian flows up the inside of the leg, in between the breasts and finishes just below the collarbone.

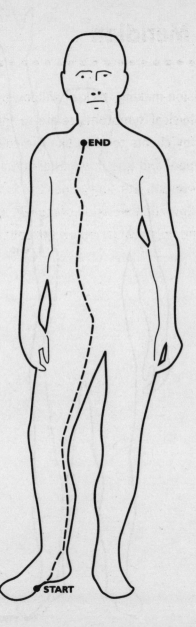

END

START

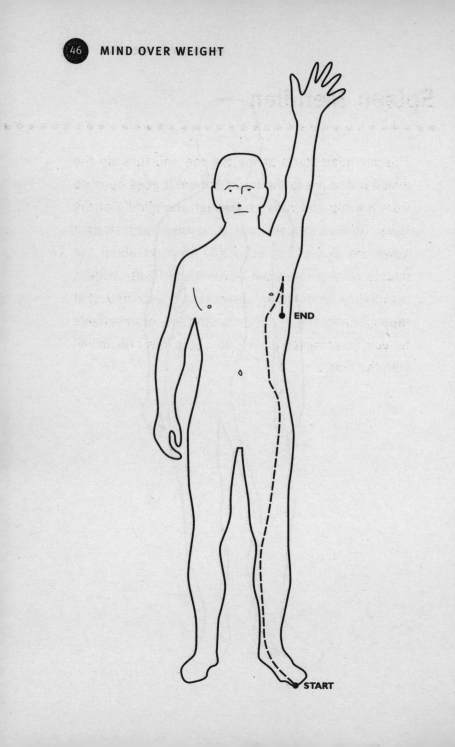

START

END

Spleen Meridian

● ●

This meridian starts at the big toe and runs up the inside of the leg to the pelvis, where it goes outward from the hip and runs up through the middle of the lower rib and into the armpit. It then runs straight down the side of the body and stops at about the middle of a bra strap. It is associated with anxiety, over-eating and eating disorders. If you find that tapping under the arm is uncomfortable or unsuitable for you, you may tap the middle of the lower rib, in line with the nipple.

Lung Meridian

• •

As its name suggests, the Lung Meridian is related to breathing disorders, asthma and nasal congestion. It increases positivity and is associated with intolerance and obsessive compulsive disorders. The Lung Meridian flows from just above the breast, up into the shoulder and down the arm ending at the thumb.

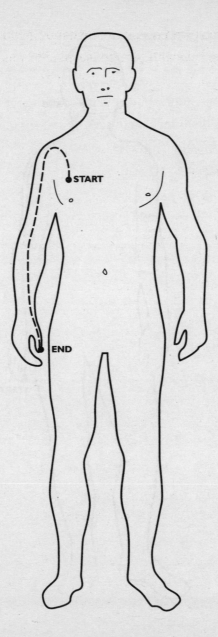

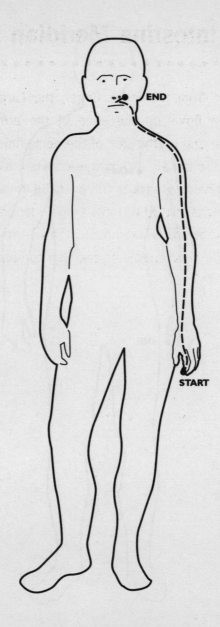

START

END

Large Intestine Meridian

Running from the index finger, the Large Intestine Meridian flows up the edge of the arm, over the shoulder and up the side of the neck, finishing at the side of the nostril. This meridian, when blocked, may cause a harking back to the past. Guilt and wellbeing are also associated with the Large Intestine Meridian, in addition to such physical ailments as bowel problems, sinus problems and skin complaints.

Circulation Sex Meridian

• •

This peculiarly named meridian is often associated with low self-esteem, jealousy, regret, sexual problems and unhappiness. Physical problems related to the Circulation Sex Meridian also encompass angina, blood pressure, circulation and heart disease. Also known as the Pericardium Meridian, it flows from the outside of the breast, up the arm, ending at the tip of the middle finger.

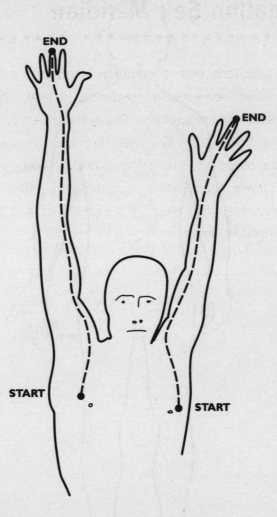

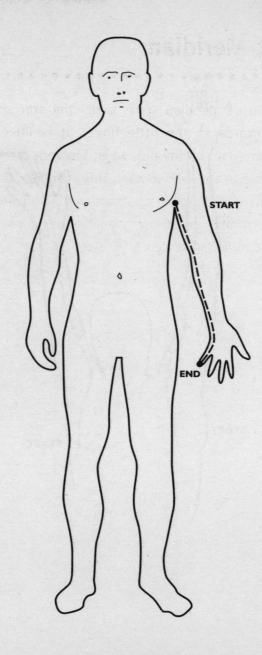

START

END

Heart Meridian

• •

The Heart Meridian starts under the arm and runs downwards to the little finger. It is linked with compassion and joy but, when blocked, can lead to loneliness and selfishness. This meridian being so closely linked to compassion and the concept of unconditional love brings credence to the concept of the heart being the centre of love.

Small Intestine Meridian

This is the meridian treated when you tap the Karate Chop point. It removes feelings of self-doubt and lack of confidence. When blocked, this meridian can cause anxiety, bad judgement and self-hate. It runs up the back of the body starting at the tip of the little finger, up the arm, across the shoulder and ends in front of the ear.

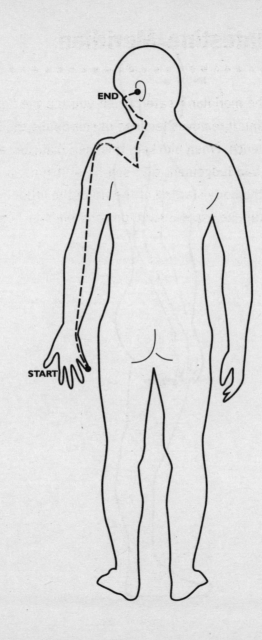

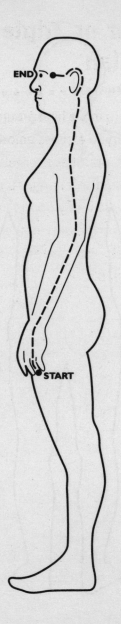

Triple Warmer or Triple Heater Meridian

This meridian helps to move heat around the body. It is related to the inability to express emotions, loneliness and resentment. If you have problems with your bladder, allergies, fluid retention, spleen or physical pain, then this meridian may be able to help. It runs from the ring finger, up the back of the arm, across the shoulder to the neck. From here it flows around the ear, ending at the temple.

UNIT 1

HOW DO I FEEL TODAY?

· ·

As a starting point, it would be useful to know how you feel today, and what characteristics you feel that you display. You will find some statements opposite and I would like you to score how much you agree or disagree with the statement. (10 would mean that you strongly agree and o would mean you strongly disagree.)

Write this score in the column marked **Score**, and we will look at the reasons later.

Statement	Score	Reason
I am not happy with my life	3	
I am self-conscious	6	Concerned over what people think of me
I am ashamed	7	Not able to control Anger, eating, or apply myself
I feel rejected	8	Kay, sex
I am insecure	8	Worried about relationship Kay going off
I am lonely	8	Travelling, when I make mistakes
I am nervous	9	Job, money, position
I am envious	9	People who succeeded
I am a failure	9	Do not have enough Cannot change
I feel vulnerable	9	Money, Job, Emotions

Statement	Score	Reason
I feel grief	2	
I feel guilt	2	
I don't fit in	6	Always felt different
I have mood swings	7	Can be happy, then very angry
I am jealous	5	
I give up too easily	8	Diets, change, Fitness, habits
I feel that life is unfair	8	Seem to get one step forward to be knocked back
I am emotional	8	Cry, Sad, Angry, Few Happys,
I have panic attacks	6	In situations of feeling I should have done something, or am late
I am angry	9	Rage at people, events, words, rebellion

Statement	Score	Reason
I am inferior	8	Feel that I am not good enough because of my faults
I feel sad	3	
I am a problem drinker	0	
I am a problem eater	8	Eat when not hungry, Eat when bored
I am very particular in my habits	2	
I do not sleep well	2	
I have poor family relations	3	
I am a worrier	7	Will turn things over and over, know at them
I am over-tidy	2	
I am a nail-biter	2	

You need to explore further any score above 5. What are the reasons behind these feelings? If you are jealous, who are you jealous of? If sad, then what are you sad about? Take your time to evaluate these questions as they will help you to identify your blocks later on in the book. Write your reasons in the column provided.

UNIT 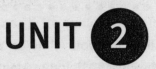 2

DISCOVERING YOUR TRUTHS

• •

Your Unconscious Mind

● ●

Your unconscious mind is an immensely powerful tool. If you doubt this statement, then consider this: if I told you that you were worthless, dumb or stupid over a period of time, how long would it take before you were emotionally affected, before your head dropped, your self-confidence started to slip away? A year ... a month ... a week?

Your unconscious mind makes up 88% of your brain's volume and keeps our hearts beating, lungs breathing and a million other things all at once. It cannot reason or learn but accepts things at face value. It does not argue but merely obeys. It is much like a computer; you programme the information in and it does as it is told.

Think about this: ideas, thoughts or instructions lodged in this part of the brain become fact. The unconscious mind accepts these as the absolute truth. But what if we were programming in all the wrong sort of information? Well, we do, all the time. *'I bet I will fail the test'* or *'I know that I will lose'* or even *'I am fat, I cannot lose weight'*, all of these statements will have a powerful impact on the unconscious mind.

Your thoughts can affect you physically; anger stimulates adrenalin, stress increases the pulse rate. Thoughts that have a high emotional charge will make their way to the unconscious mind and produce the same bodily reaction time after time. It is estimated that 80% of illness has an emotional base. In its very simplest form, negative emotions, such as stress or anxiety, can lead to ulcers, migraines and irritable bowel syndrome, but at its most powerful, the effects can be devastating.

If somebody referring to you as worthless over a long period of time leads to you feeling worthless, what if that person called you fat, chunky or porky. Even if meant as a joke, these comments can settle in the deepest recesses of your unconscious mind. When it comes to the time to lose weight, you simply cannot, your body will not allow you to *because you are fat, and that is what you are*. It has become one of your truths! It has become a barrier to weight loss. And you may have more barriers set deep within your belief system.

Your Belief System

• •

Your beliefs are your *truths*. These truths are fashioned over time by experience, those in authority or our friends and colleagues. Your belief systems are an integral part of your weight. If we both read a newspaper article, you would interpret it according to your truths, and me to mine. You may be an absolute advocate of the death penalty, whilst your friend may be vehemently opposed to it. Who is right is a matter of opinion, an opinion based on your *truths*. Importantly, these truths often lie at a deeply unconscious level.

As we discovered, your unconscious mind is a powerful tool; it can lead you to illness and even weight gain. The good news is that it can be trained. **A trained mind will set its own limits**. It will guide you in what to eat, when you need exercise and allow you to achieve your desired weight safely.

Most importantly, these things will become natural, you will want to do them because your mind is trained that way. Your truths have been rewritten. Your truths may currently be:

Fat people are happier
I cannot lose weight
I am big boned
I have a slow metabolism
etc ...

These need to be substituted with beliefs that are altogether more appropriate, with beliefs that are compatible with your target weight.

The good news is that this is not as difficult as it may sound.

Please write your target weight below.

My target weight is ...... 11st 7lbs ....

Now write the weight that you *really want to achieve*, the one that you think you never will achieve. Let's call it your *desired weight*...

My desired weight is ...... 11st 7lbs ....

Is there a difference? If so, think about why that might

be. Your truths may be blocking your ability to achieve your desired weight. It is important, therefore, that we uncover what your truths are. Your truths have become your blocks to effective weight loss.

Please now score your belief that you can achieve your *desired* weight. (Circle a figure below.)

Do Not Believe 0 1 2 3 4 5 6 7 8 9 10 **Really Believe**

It will be very difficult to achieve your desired weight if your score is below a 7. If you have no belief that you can achieve your goal, then your goal is more likely to remain out of reach.

I am now going to give you your **GOAL STATEMENT**. **It is important that you learn it and say it as often as you can, even if your belief in it is low.**

Say to yourself out loud: **'I weigh (insert *desired* weight) and that is what I weigh.'**

This is perhaps best not done in a public place, you may get some strange looks! This is your **GOAL STATEMENT**; remember it, and say it every day.

Do you believe it? Answer honestly.

I thought not.

Why not? Because in the back of your mind are all those nagging doubts, your truths, your blocks. Tick the general blocks below which apply to you:

General Blocks	Score
☑ I cannot lose weight easily	3
☐ It is impossible for me to lose weight	....
☐ I am big boned	....
☐ I have a slow metabolism	....
☑ People naturally put on weight as they grow older	4
☐ Fat people are happier	....
☑ I will not be loved if I am thin	3
☑ I will put it all back on again	6
☐ I am happy as I am	....
☐ I am this weight naturally	....
☑ I need someone to love and accept me as I am, before I can lose weight	2

●◆

General Blocks   Score

☐ Others in my family are overweight,
   it is only natural that I will be, too   ....

☑ I do not feel safe leaving my comfort zone ....2...

☐ I feel more comfortable where I am   ....

☑ I eat when I am bored   ...7...

☑ I eat when I am unhappy   ...8....

☐ I feel guilty every time I eat   ....

☑ I eat when I am anxious   ...9....

☐ I eat when I am ....

☐ I have been told that I am fat by ....
   for .... years   ....
   (insert name and number of years)

Now write your own blocks below. You really need to be honest with yourself here. If you don't list your blocks here, then it will be difficult to remove them later. You may add to the list at any time.

Your Personal Blocks   **Score**

1. I dont apply myself   8

2. I avoid working   7
    ↳ Whys

3. ~~I feel good~~ eating makes   5
    me feel better

4. ....

5. I want to be part of things   3

6. I'm Jealous of my   3
    familys lifestyle

7. I dont want to work   2

8. ....

9. ....

10. ....

Now go back over all the statements that you have ticked or added yourself, and score them on a 0–10 scale, 0 being irrelevant and 10 being very relevant. Write your score next to the statements.

UNIT 3

EMOTIONAL BARRIERS

··

Now that you have listed your blocks to weight loss, you need to discover any emotional issues that are linked to an increased awareness of your body, especially weight. A traumatic event can often trigger weight gain, or a heightened perception of your body that may manifest itself as a weight problem. Refer back to Unit 1 for clues if you need to.

Look at the example of a life chart below:

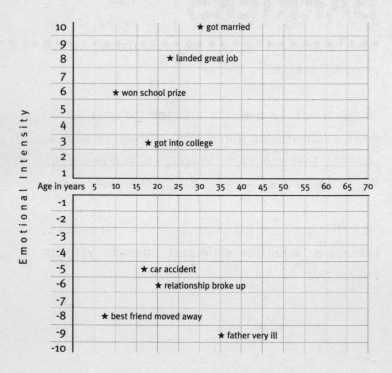

You will see that there is a scale of 10 to -10 on the left-hand side. This is the level of **emotional intensity you still feel now** about a particular incident in your life. 10 would indicate very good memories and -10 very bad ones. You will see your age go up by five years at a time from 0 to 75.

In the example above, there are several significant moments and their corresponding level of emotional intensity **which is still being felt now**. The car accident, which was suffered at the age of 16, still holds a score of -5, and the marriage at 31 still provokes a response of 10.

To create your own life chart, pinpoint at what age an event happened (or, if in doubt, estimate as near as you can). Then score it either up to +10 or down to -10. Put a cross where the age and emotional score meet.

Now fill in your own life chart overleaf, and **remember, the score is for the emotional intensity you are feeling now.**

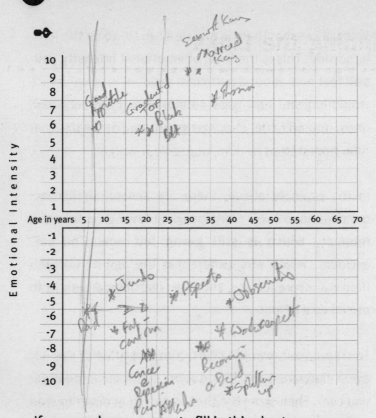

If you need more space to fill in this chart you can copy
and enlarge it.

Finding the Links

● ●

Now that you have plotted your events, draw a line from the top of the chart to the bottom, at the age that you **first** started to think about your weight.

Next, draw another line when weight issues featured heavily in your life. NB: You may only need to draw one line, but if you have weight issues on and off over varying periods of your life, then you need to draw a line through **each age that you considered weight to be an issue**.

You should now be able to see a correlation (if there is one) between significant events in your life and weight issues. This chart may show up if an event triggered weight gain or, indeed, different perceptions that you began to have about your body.

It is also worth mentioning that triggers are often at an unconscious level and therefore we may not be aware of them, because they have become our truths. It may be worth confiding in a close friend, and asking them if you changed emotionally or physically after certain events. Ask them to be honest with you but be prepared for the truth.

Please write your emotional issues below:

[Example:
*Gained weight after getting married, first few months
we argued a lot. Felt unloved.*
Car accident. Shock and trauma. Still having bad dreams.]

➥ Cancer & Depression. Panic Attacks
....

Gained weight - Good appetite
....

Married issues - Unloved
....

Splitting up unloved
....

BULLY ISSUES
....

Please score your current level of happiness (circle a
figure below):

➥

Unhappy 0 1 2 (3) 4 5 (6) 7 8 9 10 **Happy**

What would you need to do in your life to make the
score higher? Write it below. (Honestly!)

Be less bothered by them

Be more positive

More comfortable salary

Happier Homelife

Lose weight / gain john

UNIT 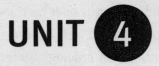 4

CRAVINGS

So far, we have worked at identifying your blocks to weight loss, and any emotional barriers you may have to achieving your desired weight. Now we are going to focus our attentions on cravings. Refer back to Unit 1 for clues if you need to.

List all the foods that you have cravings for:

●◆

...... Sweet things ....

...... Food in general ....

....

....

....

Is there a specific time of day that you get these cravings? ●◆ Yes/No

If yes, does that time of day correspond with an event that still causes you emotional disturbance? (*E.g. a car crash at 11.00am coincides with craving for chocolate at this time of day.*)

- Evenings / Nights

Telley or computer or reading

Afternoons — habitual snack

Continual eating

What emotions are you feeling when you get the craving? (*E.g. Insecure, bored, tired ...*)

- Bored, Tired

Insecure, Anxious

Worried nervous

If you gave up this craving, what would be the good points?

➤
I would lose weight
Not feel bloated e
unhealthy
Not feel guilty

If you gave up this craving, what would be the bad points? (This is a lot harder, but what would you miss?)

➤
Tastes / flavours
Endorphines
Feeling better

What physical symptoms do you feel when you start to get the craving? (*E.g. Taste at the back of the throat, butterflies in stomach, etc.*)

➡ Need to eat. Some hungry?

Unable to settle

If these symptoms were linked to a specific event, what would that event be? (When have you felt these symptoms before?)

➡ Unloved?

Concern over work / or life.

To much work to do

Worried about what people think

UNIT 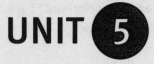 5

SELF-IMAGE

....

Imagine yourself at your desired weight. Go on, really visualise it. Is it easy or really hard? If it is really hard, then why is that so? Refer back to Unit 1 for clues if you need to.

What do you look like? Are you confident and happy? Describe yourself below. For instance, would you be more attractive to the opposite sex and, if so, would that be a good or bad thing?

Confident, strong, lean
fit, able to make good
decisions, more patient,
calm, better father
Relaxed e balanced
More dynamic

What would be the good things about achieving your desired weight? List them below.

➡ Not feeling bloated/ill

Less injurys

More able to do exercise

Faster @ running

Food is controlled not controlling

Stronger in mind & body

Live longer

What would be the bad things about achieving your desired weight? Has anything happened to you before at this weight? For instance, you may have had a traumatic event whilst at your desired weight. List them below.

Depression, Panic Attacks
? Anger at something ?
? Joanna ?
Cancer
Relationship issues
Car accidents ?
Father / family issues
Aspects ?

What would other people say? List all of those who would be genuinely happy for you.

➡ .... Lost weight ....

.... Looking good ....

.... Well done ....

.... Family, friends, colleagues ....

....

....

....

....

....

....

....

Now list those who would not be happy if you achieved your desired weight. Are these people important in your life?

•◦

....

....

....

....

....

....

....

....

....

....

....

These exercises may have given you some clues to issues
you may have regarding weight loss. Are they linked to an
event or person? Write any specific issues below.

Cancer

Father / home

Work concerns — Stress
— Anger/Fear

View of myself

Depression

Panic Attacks

End of Relationships

Inability to maintain relationships

UNIT 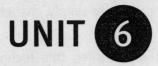 6

HOW IS IT DONE?

• •

I will now show you the straightforward, yet remarkable technique that can, quite simply, change your life!

As I have outlined earlier, this technique is called Emotional Freedom Technique, or EFT for short, and was developed by Gary Craig. He simplified it and made it available to all, an extremely generous gesture once you realise the impact EFT can have on our everyday lives.

The Science Bit!

We have already looked briefly at the job meridians perform — carrying electrical energy around the body.

If you take the back off of your radio or hi-fi and poke around with a big screwdriver, the chances are that you may cause a short circuit and this may lead to loss of signal, fuzzy sound or disrupted quality.

Your body also has electrical circuits. That is how your heart beats, why we get static electricity and how we feel pain, because it is electrically transmitted; but these electrical circuits can also become short circuited. Modern medicine actually measures electrical activity when carrying out ECGs (electrocardiographs). When our energy stops flowing, we die. It is as simple as that; ask your doctor.

The Discovery Statement

• •

Gary Craig realised that 'the cause of all negative emotion is a disruption in the body's energy system'. I described earlier how 80% of illness is emotionally based. Therefore, 80% of illness is caused by a disruption in the body's energy system. On top of this, your negative emotions about weight, your blocks, are caused, yes, by a disruption in the body's energy system.

Distressing Memory = Short Circuit = Negative Emotion

Straighten out the short circuit and the negative emotion goes away and, with it, the illness, blocks or barriers that are inhibiting you.

Simply put, energy flows around the body like a river, but that energy can get blocked, in the same way as a log can block a river. The energy cannot continue to flow until the blockage is removed. It will either build up or take an alternate course. This can cause a 'short circuit' in the energy system that needs to be corrected. To correct it, all you need to do is tap the meridian at a specified point whilst focusing on the problem.

Right now, you are probably thinking, 'Come off it, it cannot be that simple.' But I will *prove* it to you. You do not even have to believe it, it will work anyway. The technique takes 10 minutes to learn.

Your Goal Statement

Remember this from earlier? You should be saying it every day by now. If not, start now, as it is an important part of the process. This is going to be your daily affirmation. Make no mistake, affirmations used properly are your most powerful tool to weight loss or self-improvement.

Say out loud:

'I weigh (insert desired weight) and that is what I weigh.'

Now score your belief in your ability to achieve this:

Do Not Believe 0 1 2 3 4 5 6 7 8 9 10 Really Believe

Wouldn't it be nice to be able to increase that score, to increase your belief that you can achieve your desired weight? Well, that is exactly what we are going to do.

The Technique

• •

At first, the steps may appear long-winded or cumbersome, but as you become acquainted with them, a complete round will only take about a minute or less.

The technique consists of four stages and is known as the EFT sandwich.

1. **The Setup**
2. **The Sequence** (bread)
3. **The Gamut Procedure** (cheese)
4. **The Sequence Repeated** (bread)

As mentioned earlier, you will need to focus in on the problem whilst tapping the points listed below. When going through this process, it is best to keep the following guidelines in mind:

• If any of the points feel nicer than others, it may be worth while tapping these a little longer, for as long as you want; in fact, you cannot overtap.

• If any point feels sore or really hurts, try switching to the other side of the body, or just touching the point for two breaths without tapping.

• Your body may react in different ways, so do not be alarmed if something out of the ordinary happens. You may be opening meridians that have not flowed properly for some time, and that can feel strange.

• After doing this procedure for the first time, I would recommend that you give yourself two or three days before trying it again. This will give your body time to settle.

1. THE SETUP

To achieve success, you need to prepare your unconscious mind, and that includes neutralising blocks to healing. This is done in **The Setup**.

Decide which hand you would feel most comfortable tapping with — if you are right-handed, this will probably be your right hand, and vice versa.

Now look at your non-tapping hand, palm upwards. Locate the edge of your hand in-between the wrist and base of your little finger. This is the point where you would 'karate chop' something if you so desired! It is therefore called the Karate Chop or KC point (see the diagram on page 121).

Remind yourself of your goal statement.

Say out loud the following statements whilst tapping the KC point on one hand with the four fingers of the other hand.

- 'Even though it will never be possible for me to achieve my goal statement, I want to deeply and completely accept myself.'

- 'Even if it unsafe for me to achieve my goal statement, I want to deeply and completely accept myself.'

- 'Even if it is unsafe for others for me to achieve my goal statement, I want to deeply and completely accept myself.'

- 'Even though I have unique blocks stopping me from achieving my goal statement, I want to deeply and completely accept myself.'

- 'Even though I don't deserve to achieve my goal statement, I want to deeply and completely accept myself.'

As you said those statements, did any of them touch a nerve or 'hit the spot'?

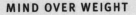

If so, write the statement here:

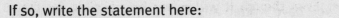

. . . .

. . . .

. . . .

Is there anything that you think you ought to have said? ➤ Yes/No

If so, write it here:
(The Setup statement should begin **'Even though I ...'**
and finish with **' ... I want to deeply and completely
accept myself.'**)

➤

. . . .

. . . .

. . . .

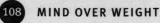

If you have written any further statements, then say these three times each whilst tapping the KC point with the four fingers of the other hand.

2: THE SEQUENCE

• •

You now need to tap all of the points whilst reminding yourself what you are tapping for, in this case your **GOAL STATEMENT**. Say out loud *'Goal Statement'* as you tap each point, as this is what you want to improve. **This is your Reminder Statement.**

You will now find a series of diagrams on the following pages, which will show you exactly which points you need to tap. It does not matter what side of the body you use, or indeed if you switch sides whilst in the middle of the sequence. Tapping should be done fairly firmly but not enough to bruise yourself! If a point hurts, instead of tapping just hold the point for two breaths. If you physically cannot tap a point then do not worry: you could imagine tapping it or miss it out altogether. You should tap about 7 times fairly quickly, whilst saying your reminder statement.

| **EB** **Eyebrow** | At beginning of eyebrow at top of nose. | Use the index finger and middle finger to tap this point. |

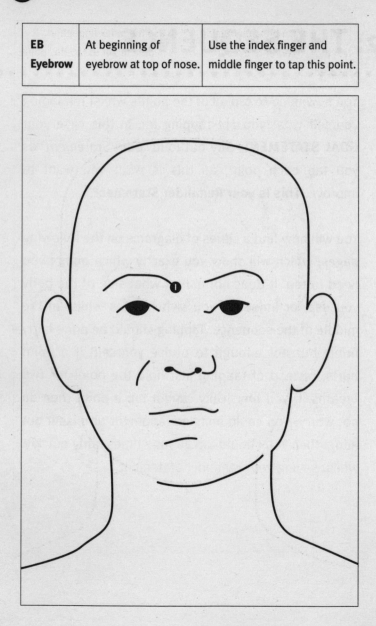

EC Eye Corner	On bone on outside corner of eye.	Use the index finger and middle finger to tap this point.

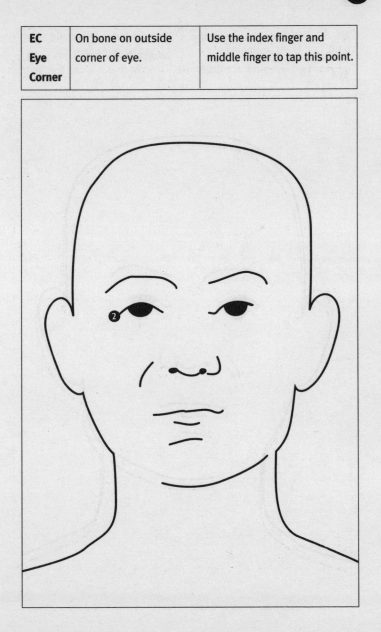

UE Under Eye	On bone just under the eye.	Use the index finger and middle finger to tap this point.

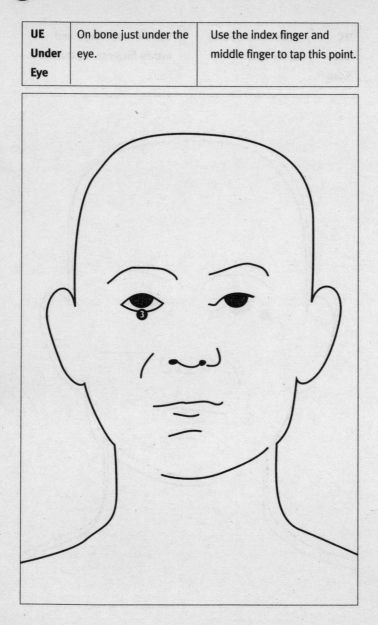

UN **Under** **Nose**	Between nose and upper lip.	Use the index finger and middle finger to tap this point.

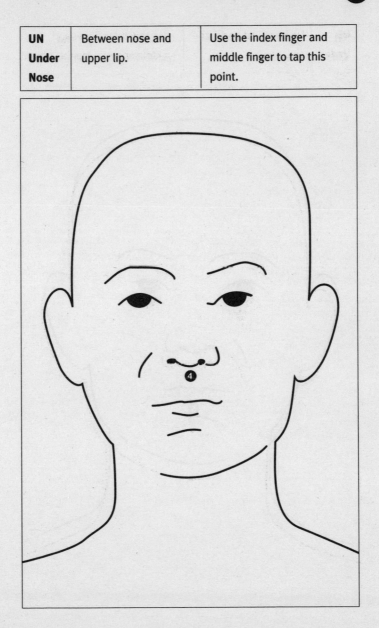

CH Chin	Centre of chin under lower lip.	Use the index finger and middle finger to tap this point.

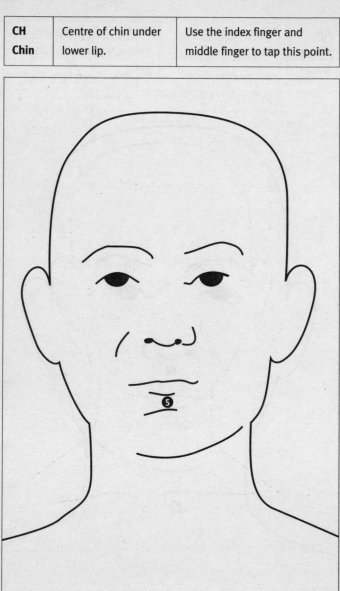

CB Collarbone	Place finger on collarbone. Move it into centre of body until you reach the corner.	Use all four fingers to tap the corner of the collarbone, fairly hard if you can.

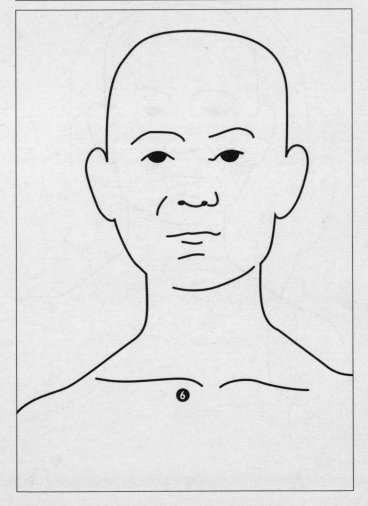

UA Under Arm	Under the arm approx. 4ins below armpit, in line with the nipple.	Use a flat palm to 'lightly slap' this point.

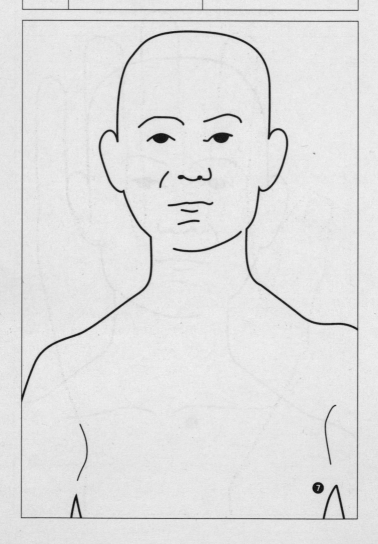

TH Thumb	Outside edge of thumb at base of nail.	Use the index finger and middle finger to tap this point.

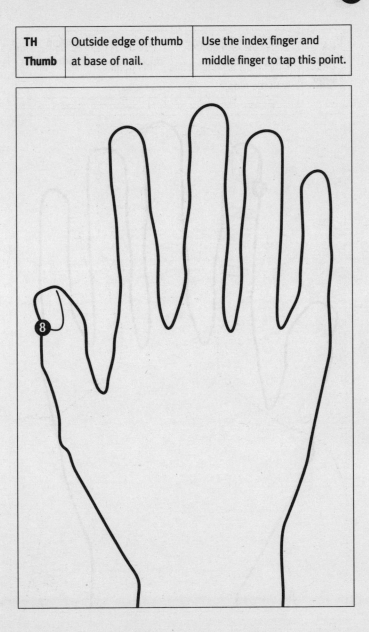

IF Index Finger	At base of nail on side facing thumb.	Use the index finger and middle finger to tap this point.

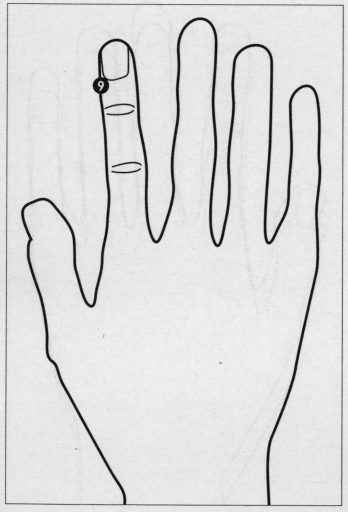

MF Middle Finger	At base of nail on side facing thumb.	Use the index finger and middle finger to tap this point.

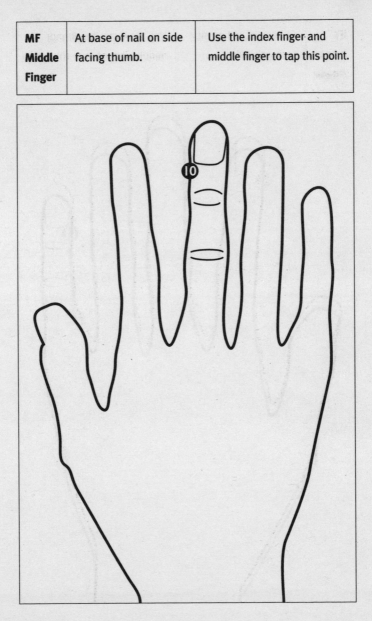

LF **Little** **Finger**	At base of nail on side facing thumb.	Use the index finger and middle finger to tap this point.

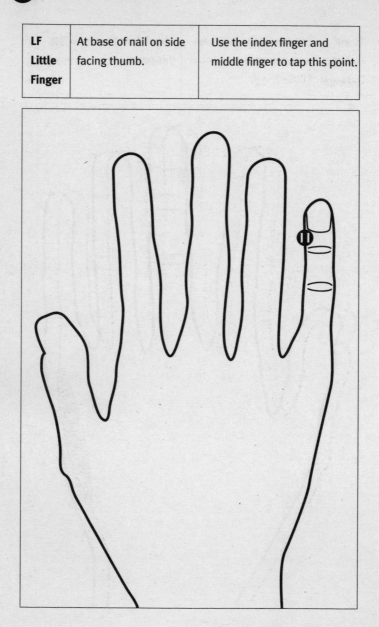

KC **Karate** **Chop**	Outside of hand between top of wrist bone and base of little finger.	Use all four fingers to tap this point.

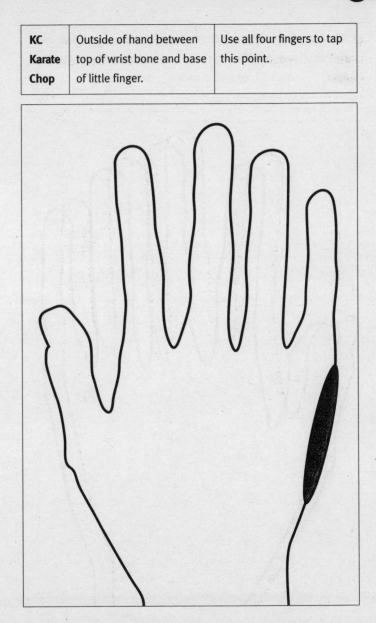

GS **Gamut** **Spot**	Back of hand, in-between ring and little finger knuckles, about 1in back up hand.	Use the index finger and middle finger to tap this point.

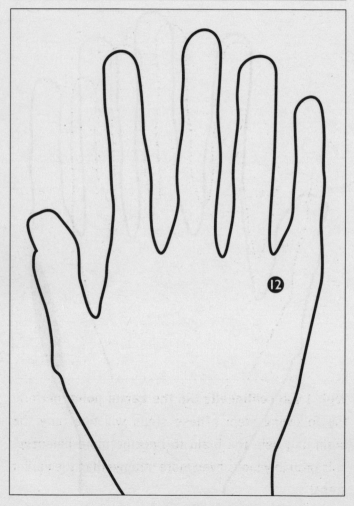

3: THE GAMUT PROCEDURE

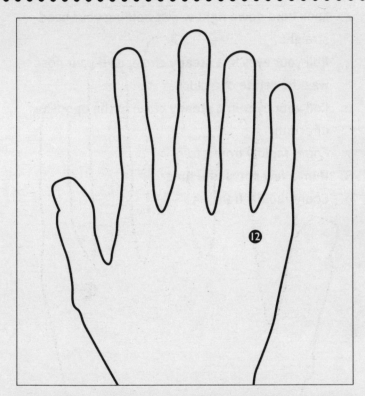

Whilst you continually tap the gamut point, perform the following steps. These steps will fine tune the brain and help the brain to become more balanced. This probably looks even more strange than the earlier steps!

1. Close your eyes
2. Open your eyes
3. Look hard down left whilst holding your head straight
4. Look hard down right whilst holding your head straight
5. Roll your eyes in a **steady** circle, as if your nose was the centre of a clock
6. Roll your eyes in a **steady** circle in the opposite direction
7. Count rapidly from 1 to 5
8. Hum a few notes of a tune
9. Count rapidly from 1-5

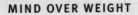

4: THE SEQUENCE REPEATED

Now repeat The Sequence, working through all the individual treatment points, from The Eyebrow to The Gamut Spot.

That is the end of this part of the technique. So how have you done? Repeat out loud your goal statement:

'I weigh (insert *desired* weight) and that is what I weigh.'

Now score your belief in your ability to achieve this:

Do Not Believe 0 1 2 3 4 5 6 7 8 9 10 **Really Believe**

Has it increased? If so, by how much?

Repeat the entire procedure again, **but you will not need to redo the Gamut Procedure** until your score is raised significantly.

In the unlikely event of your score not increasing, try changing rooms or drinking water before trying again, or see the **Troubleshooting** section at the back of this book.

UNIT 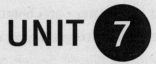 7

BREATHING EXERCISES

•••

These exercises are a useful tool to aid the meridian flow, relax and invigorate. The Collarbone Breathing exercise will help you if you are having trouble shifting your score to any significant degree. You should not need this, but if you do, then perform this routine before you start your treatment. The Balanced Breathing and Calming Breath are relaxation techniques that you could easily utilise in a quiet moment before treatment.

Collarbone Breathing

• •

The Collarbone Breathing exercise will help you if you are having trouble shifting your score to any significant degree.

This technique utilises 40 breathing and tapping movements. During the exercise, keep your arms away from your body so that only your fingertips and knuckles touch your body.

1. Place two fingers of your right hand on your right collarbone point, and with two fingers of your left hand tap the gamut point on your right hand continuously whilst you:
2. Breathe in halfway and hold for 7 taps
3. Breathe all the way in and hold for 7 taps
4. Breathe out halfway and hold for 7 taps
5. Breathe all the way out and hold for 7 taps
6. Breathe normally for 7 taps
7. Now place the two fingers from your right hand on your left collarbone and repeat
8. Next, bend the fingers on your right hand and place the knuckles on your right collarbone and repeat

9. Now place the knuckles of your right hand on your left collarbone and repeat

10. You have now done half the procedure; do the same routine as in points 1–6 above, but this time using the left hand to touch the collarbone

Balanced Breathing

• •

This is a wonderful exercise, especially if you are feeling particularly stressed or 'unbalanced'. To my mind, it is the best breathing exercise bar none.

1. Sit upright in a chair
2. Cross your feet over
3. Cross your arms over in the opposite direction to your feet
4. Turn palms in towards each other and hold hands (your wrists should be crossed)
5. Breathe in through your nose with the tip of your tongue on the roof of your mouth (this ensures that two powerful channels, the Central and Governing vessels, are connected)
6. Breathe out through your mouth with your tongue lying flat. As you breathe out, think 'BALANCE'
7. Continue for 2 minutes only

Diaphragmatic Breathing — The Calming Breath

• •

Breathing solely from the diaphragm needs practice. You need to spend a few minutes each day for one week until you are able to use this method whilst sitting, lying, standing or walking. As soon as you start to feel any stress or anxiety, begin to use the diaphragmatic breathing, this will immediately have a calming effect and will, in most instances, avert the anxiety and stress. It is no use waiting until the stress reaches its height; it needs to be practised at the beginning to prevent the stress from building and becoming unmanageable.

1. Place the flat of your right hand on your diaphragm (the top of your stomach), left hand on chest

2. Looking down, begin by taking a 'normal' breath in and, as you do so, notice the movement of your hands as you breathe in and out

3. Now, taking another breath in, physically push out the diaphragm, making sure that the left hand – on the chest – does not move; you are only concerned with the movement of the diaphragm

4. As you breathe out, you should feel your right hand return to its original position

5. Repeat

If you find **Diaphragmatic Breathing** difficult, here are a couple of ideas that may help you.

• Imagine that you have a piece of string, about 10in long coming out of your diaphragm.

Now imagine holding that piece of string about 10in away from your body, begin moving that string away from your body very, very slowly whilst you take a slow, deep breath in through your nose. And, as you are breathing in, allow your diaphragm to come out with that string.

After counting for '3 elephants' (as in '1 elephant, 2 elephants, 3 elephants ...') — slowly let that piece of string gently move back towards your body, letting the string hang loosely, and you'll find that you are releasing that 'calming' breath from your body nice and slowly whilst you are letting the string return back to its loose position.

• Try this breathing exercise using a straw. Breathe in and out through the straw.

Initially, watch yourself in front of a mirror. If the left hand (on the chest) moves, you are doing it incorrectly. It is then easier to practise whilst lying down and I suggest that you practise for a few minutes when you wake up in the morning and a few minutes before going to sleep at night.

At first, you will probably find that it is only possible to take two or three diaphragmatic breaths before needing to gasp and maybe take a few deep breaths. Don't worry, this is quite normal and you will find that, with practice, you will be able to breathe diaphragmatically for a few minutes at a time.

Many people practise this form of breathing for a couple of days and think that is all they need to do. It does need practice so that it can be called upon to be used automatically and efficiently as and when needed.

If you experience any discomfort or dizziness, stop immediately and ask an expert for help, as you might not be doing the breathing correctly.

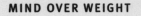

UNIT 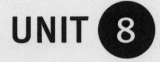 8

CLEARING THE BLOCKS TO WEIGHT LOSS

Now that your belief that you can achieve your desired weight has improved, you need to start breaking down your blocks to weight loss. These are the blocks that you listed earlier in Unit 2.

This is done using the four stages of treatment in Unit 6:

1. **The Setup**
2. **The Sequence**
3. **The Gamut Procedure**
4. **The Sequence Repeated**

Now turn back to the list of blocks that you made in Unit 2 and select one to erase now. For the purpose of this exercise, I will use 'I have a slow metabolism'.

Now score your belief in your statement:

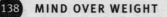

Do Not Believe 0 1 2 3 4 5 6 7 8 9 10 **Really Believe**

1. The Setup

• •

Tapping the KC spot repeat:

'Even though *I have a slow metabolism*, I want to deeply and completely accept myself.'

Yours may be:

'Even though *people put on weight as they get older*, I want to deeply and completely accept myself.'
or
'Even though *I am this weight naturally*, I want to deeply and completely accept myself.'

2: The Sequence

• •

Now choose a reminder statement to say as you tap on each point. I am going to say 'slow metabolism'.

Now tap on all of the treatment points whilst repeating your reminder statement. Really tune into, and think about your block.

Remember:

• If any of the points feel nicer than others, it may be worthwhile tapping these a little longer, for as long as you want, in fact; you cannot overtap.

• If any point feels sore or really hurts, try switching to the other side of the body, or just holding the point for two breaths.

• Your body may react in different ways, so do not be alarmed if something out of the ordinary happens. You may be opening meridians that have not flowed properly for some time, and that can feel strange.

3: The Gamut Procedure

Now perform the Gamut Procedure as described in Unit 6 on page 123/124.

4: The Sequence Repeated

Repeat the sequence.

Now score your belief in your block:

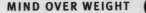

Do Not Believe 0 1 2 3 4 5 6 7 8 9 10 Really Believe

Has it gone down? Do the whole treatment again, *although you need not do the Gamut Procedure again*, until you get your score as low as you possibly can.

Now repeat this process for each of your blocks. I realise that this may take a little time, but you are eradicating a lifetime's worth of blocks and replacing them with one — your Goal Statement.

If, like many of us, you have a great long list that keeps growing as you identify more blocks, then just do two, three or as many as you can cope with, each day. You will notice that as you eradicate them one by one, you will start to feel better in yourself, your confidence may improve and you may begin to feel more relaxed.

When you are happy that you have cleared these blocks, then please proceed.

UNIT 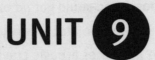 9

CLEARING CRAVINGS

• •

Wouldn't it be great if, every time you had a craving for your favourite food, you could get rid of that feeling by tapping just one or two points? This will be the goal for this section. To get rid of a basic craving you should only really need to do **The Setup** and **The Sequence**. If this does not work, then put in **The Gamut Procedure** as well, but you usually won't have to.

This section will work best if you actually have the craving right now. If you cannot get your score for the craving up to at least a 7, then you really need to wait until you can get a high enough score to treat it effectively.

The important thing about this particular use of The Sequence is for you to try to identify a point or maybe two points that really work for you; a point that you can feel the craving go as you tap it. This may take a few rounds for you to identify, so do not worry if you do not get it the first time through.

Think of your favourite food. Imagine the smell. If you have some available now then go and get some. Hold it, look at it, feel it; now how good would it be to taste? Score the craving now:

●◆

No Craving   0 1 2 3   4   5 6 7 8 9 10 Must Eat It!

1: The Setup

Tapping the KC spot repeat:

**'Even though *I have this craving for*.................,
I want to deeply and completely accept myself.'**

Repeat this twice more.

2: The Sequence

As a reminder statement, as you tap on each point say
out loud *'this craving'*.

Now tap on all of the points listed above whilst
repeating your reminder statement. Really tune into
your craving.

Remember:

• If any of the points feel nicer than others, it may be worthwhile tapping these a little longer, for as long as you want, in fact; you cannot overtap.

• If any point feels sore or really hurts, try switching to the other side of the body, or just holding the point for two breaths.

• Your body may react in different ways, so do not be alarmed if something out of the ordinary happens. You may be opening meridians that have not flowed properly for some time, and that can feel strange.

3: The Gamut Procedure

• •

Only do this if the sequence is not working.

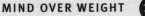

4: The Sequence Repeated

Repeat the sequence.

Score the craving now:

No Craving   0 1 2 3 4 5 6 7 8 9 10 **Must Eat It!**

Has it gone down? Do the whole treatment again, *although you need not do the Gamut Procedure again*, until you get your score as low as you possibly can.

Every time you get a craving, do this procedure; it should take the craving away. Practise until you have it well rehearsed. **The Setup** and **The Sequence** should only take you about 30–45 seconds in all.

If you have identified just one point that works alone, then you only need to tap this. This is your 'emergency stop' point. Often, just tapping one or two **'emergency stop'** points will be enough to reduce a craving. This will only take a few seconds, as opposed to 30–45 seconds for a complete round of **The Sequence.**

UNIT 10

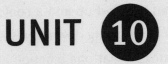

CLEARING EMOTIONAL BARRIERS

This is probably the hardest to do because emotional issues are often jumbled up into a confusing mess. It is made easier by breaking down any issues into easy-to-manage chunks. Treat one emotion at a time, fear, shame, anger, jealousy, etc.

Under the section marked **Finding the Links** in Unit 3, I asked you to write down any emotional issues. Turn back to that section now and choose an issue. Think about it from the beginning of the incident. Run it through in your mind. When you feel your emotional intensity start to rise (the emotional intensity is the feeling inside that may manifest itself as anger, shame, etc.), then identify what the emotion is.

What is the emotion? Write it here:
(For example, *Fear, Embarrassment*, etc.)

•➔

. . . .

. . . .

Is the emotion aimed at the situation, yourself, another
person, an object or anything else? Write it here:
(For example, *Fear of the knife, Ashamed of my body,
Embarrassed by his attention*, etc.)

✒

. . . .

. . . .

. . . .

So, by now, you should have an emotion and probably
a target for that emotion.

Now score the emotional intensity you feel. You may
need to really imagine the event to get your score up
as high as possible:

✒

No Emotion 0 1 2 3 4 5 6 7 8 9 10 Extreme Emotion

For emotional issues, you will generally need to go through all four stages of treatment:

1. The Setup
2. The Sequence
3. The Gamut Procedure
4. The Sequence Repeated

1: The Setup

• •

Tapping the KC spot, and using your own Setup phrases, repeat three times:

'Even though *I was embarrassed by his attention***, I want to deeply and completely accept myself.'**
Yours may be:
'Even though *I was ashamed***, I want to deeply and completely accept myself.'**
or
'Even though *I hated her for what she was doing to me***, I want to deeply and completely accept myself.'**

2: The Sequence

Now choose a reminder statement to say as you tap on each point. I am going to say 'embarrassed'.

Now tap on all of the points of The Sequence whilst repeating your reminder statement. Really tune into, and imagine, the events that led you to feel this emotion.

Remember:
• If any of the points feel nicer than others, it may be worthwhile tapping these a little longer, for as long as you want, in fact; you cannot overtap.

• If any point feels sore or really hurts, try switching to the other side of the body, or just holding the point for two breaths.

• Your body may react in different ways, so do not be alarmed if something out of the ordinary happens. You may be opening meridians that have not flowed properly for some time, and that can feel strange.

3: The Gamut Procedure

● ●

Now perform The Gamut Procedure.

4: The Sequence Repeated

● ●

Repeat the sequence.

Now score your emotional intensity again:

●◆

No Emotion 0 1 2 3 4 5 6 7 8 9 10 Extreme Emotion

The score should have gone down. If not drink some water, change rooms and try again. If you still have no movement, then see the **Troubleshooting** section at the back of the book.

Has it gone down? Do the whole treatment again, *although you need not do the Gamut Procedure again*, until you get your score as low as you possibly can. **The emotion may have been replaced by another. If so, do not be alarmed, just treat each emotion as it** arises, until you can think through the entire sequence of events in your mind without any emotional intensity.

Treat each particular aspect of the event in exactly the same way until it has no emotional hold over you. You may find yourself thinking about it less, or seeing things from a different perspective. There is no blueprint, it affects us all differently.

Repeat all of the steps for each of your emotional barriers.

UNIT 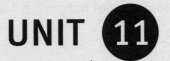 11

FINDING PERSONAL HAPPINESS

Under the section **Finding the Links** in Unit 3, I asked you to score your level of happiness. I would like you to do it again.

Please score your current level of happiness:

•◇

Unhappy   0   1   2   3   4   5   6   7   8   9   10   **Happy**

•◇

. . . .
. . . .

What would you need to do in your life to make the score higher? Write it below. (Honestly!) Refer back to Unit 1 for clues if you need to.

Has it changed from your earlier answer, now that you have done most of the exercises in this workbook? If not, you need to treat these in the same way as emotional barriers in the previous section.

For example:
I need a new challenge
I am unsatisfied at work
I have no real friends

But you need to ask yourself Why? Why? Why? Keep asking and keep getting the answers until you peel away all of the layers of the problem.

For example:
I am unsatisfied at work.

Why?

I hate my boss.

Why?

Because his job should have been mine.

Why wasn't it?

Because I am not good enough to do his job.

Aha!

1: The Setup

• •

Your Setup statement would then be:

'Even though *I am not good enough in my work* ...'

So question the answers you gave when I asked you what you needed to do to raise your happiness score. Keep asking yourself why. Peel back the layers to get to the core issue.

2: The Sequence

• •

Now choose a reminder statement to say as you tap on each point.

Now tap on all of the treatment points listed above whilst repeating your reminder statement. Really tune into, and imagine, the events that led you to feel this emotion.

Remember:

• If any of the points feel nicer than others, it may be worthwhile tapping these a little longer, for as long as you want, in fact; you cannot overtap.

- If any point feels sore or really hurts, try switching to the other side of the body, or just holding the point for two breaths.

- Your body may react in different ways, so do not be alarmed if something out of the ordinary happens. You may be opening meridians that have not flowed properly for some time, and that can feel strange.

3: The Gamut Procedure

Now perform The Gamut Procedure.

4: The Sequence Repeated

Now repeat the sequence.

Now give it a score:

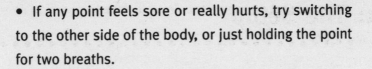

Unhappy 0 1 2 3 4 5 6 7 8 9 10 **Happy**
The score should have gone up. If not, drink some water, change rooms and try again. If you still have no

improvement, then see the **Troubleshooting** section at the back of the book.

Has it gone up? Do the whole treatment again, *although you need not do the Gamut Procedure again*, until you get your score as high as you possibly can.

The reason for your unhappiness may have been replaced by another. If so, do not be alarmed, just treat each reason as it arises.

UNIT 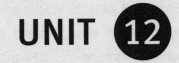 12

YOUR SELF-IMAGE

• •

Do you remember that in Unit 5 I asked you to imagine yourself at your desired weight? Was it hard for you? Did you write down why? If so, remind yourself by writing down the reasons here.

•◆

. . . .

. . . .

. . . .

Please score your current level of satisfaction with the way you look:

•◆

Dissatisfied 0 1 2 3 4 5 6 7 8 9 10 **Satisfied**

. . . .

. . . .

. . . .

What would be the bad things about achieving your desired weight? For instance, would you be more attractive to the opposite sex and, if so, would that be a good or bad thing? Has anything happened to you before whilst you were at your desired weight? List your responses below:

....

....

....

....

Now list those who would not be happy if you achieved your desired weight. Are these people important in your life?

....

....

....

What are the bad points about how you will look at your desired weight?

➡

....

....

....

You will see that I have focused on all the negative points about your self-image at your desired weight. These can form powerful blocks to achieving success. They must be cleared using EFT. Use all four stages to eradicate all of these blocks.

For example:

1: The Setup

'Even though *my husband likes me big* ...'
'Even though *fat people are happier*'
'Even though *I may attract the wrong sort of partner* ...'

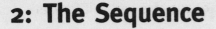

2: The Sequence

Choose a reminder statement to say as you tap on each point.

Now tap on all of the points listed above whilst repeating your reminder statement. Really tune into, and imagine, the events that led you to feel this emotion.

Remember:

• If any of the points feel nicer than others, it may be worthwhile tapping these a little longer, for as long as you want, in fact; you cannot overtap.

• If any point feels sore or really hurts, try switching to the other side of the body, or just holding the point for two breaths.

• Your body may react in different ways, so do not be alarmed if something out of the ordinary happens. You may be opening meridians that have not flowed properly for some time, and that can feel strange.

3: The Gamut Procedure

Now perform The Gamut Procedure.

4: The Sequence Repeated

Repeat the sequence.

Now score your self-image again:

Dissatisfied 0 1 2 3 4 5 6 7 8 9 10 **Satisfied**

The score should have gone up. If not drink some water, change rooms and try again. If you still have no improvement, then see the **Troubleshooting** section at the back of the book.

Has it gone up? Do the whole treatment again, *although you need not do the Gamut Procedure again*, until you get your score as high as you possibly can.

The reason for your dissatisfaction may have been

replaced by another. If so, do not be alarmed, just treat each emotion as it arises. You need to clear each of these reasons before moving on.

UNIT 13

MEASURING THE CHANGE

• •

By now you should have tackled all of the blocks and barriers to your achieving your desired weight. **Without sneaking a look at your earlier answers,** I would like you to fill in this table again. Score each statement from 0 to 10 in the **Score 1** column. A zero score would mean that you completely disagree and 10 would mean that you completely agree.

Statement	Score 1	Score 2	Reason
I am not happy with my life			
I am self-conscious			
I am ashamed			
I feel rejected			
I am insecure			
I am lonely			
I am nervous			
I am envious			
I am a failure			
I feel vulnerable			

Statement	Score 1	Score 2	Reason
I feel grief			
I feel guilt			
I don't fit in			
I have mood swings			
I am jealous			
I give up too easily			
I feel that life is unfair			
I am emotional			
I have panic attacks			
I am angry			

●◆

Statement	Score 1	Score 2	Reason
I am inferior			
I feel sad			
I am a problem drinker			
I am a problem eater			
I am very particular in my habits			
I do not sleep well			
I have poor family relations			
I am a worrier			
I am over-tidy			
I am a nail-biter			

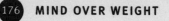
Now turn back to Unit 1 and put your scores from there in the **Score 2** column. You can now compare the two scores. Any scores that are still high need to have the reason explored. Remember back to Unit 11 when I was telling you to question your feelings, and ask yourself why, and peel back the outer layers until you get to the core. You can then treat the issues using EFT.

UNIT 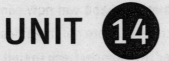 14

OVER TO YOU

....

Say to yourself out loud: **'I weigh (insert *desired* weight) and that is what I weigh.'**

Now score your belief in that statement:

Do Not Believe 0 1 2 3 4 5 6 7 8 9 10 **Really Believe**

Do two rounds of EFT using **'Even though I will never achieve my goal statement, I want to deeply and completely accept myself'** and score again.

You should by now be **very** familiar with your goal statement, and saying it every day. Does it feel as impossible now as it did at the beginning of the book? I would certainly hope not!

Now all you need to do is tune in and listen to your body. At some point in our lives, we have all eaten something, and as we are eating it we are saying to ourselves, 'I don't know why I am eating this, I do not want it.' You may find your desire for the healthier option improves. You may change your shopping and eating habits. You may even find that you would prefer to walk rather than take the car.

All this may be happening at a very subtle unconscious level, where it belongs. After all, this is where most of your blocks and barriers have been operating. Continue doing the exercises as and when the need arises, if your confidence is starting to slip, whenever you get a craving or whenever you discover a new block. The process is ever evolving.

THE MERIDIANS, POINTS AND HOW THEY AFFECT YOU

● ●

Meridian	Point	When Blocked	When Tapped	Psychological	Physical
Bladder	EB	Increase of fear and intimidation	Increases courage and releases fear	Courage, energy, fear, free expression, forgetfulness, frustration, impatience, inhibition, lethargy, restlessness, short-term memory recall, trauma, thinking processes	Automatic nervous system, lower back pain, bones, ears, hair loss, head, incontinence, osteoporosis, parasympathetic nervous system, prostate, spinal column, sympathetic nervous system, teeth, urinatory system, vertigo
Gall Bladder	EC	Depletes energy	Increases determination, and removes lethargy	Calm, courage, determination, indecision, clarity of mind	Lack of bile, fat digestion, eye problems, lack of flexibility, gall bladder, gall stones, headaches, indigestion, stiff joints, painful joints, migraine, stiff/painful muscles, poor stamina, stiff neck, stiffness, tendons/ligaments

Meridian	Point	When Blocked	When Tapped	Psychological	Physical
Stomach	UE	Muddled thinking	Releases indecisive emotions and helps thinking process	Addictions, anxiety, confused thought, deprivation, disorientation, dogmatic thinking, harmony, indecisiveness, intuition, obsessiveness	Appetite disorders, anorexia nervosa, breasts, chewing mouth and lips, upper digestive passages, endometriosis, fibroids, flesh, hiatus hernia, indigestion, mastitis, menstrual problems, nausea, ovaries, prolapses, sickness, sleep cycles, stomach, vomiting, weight problems
Governing	UN	Introvertedness	Removes shyness and helps communication skills	Communication, embarrassment, introvertedness, panic, relationships, sex problems, shyness, worry	Backache, nasal congestion, epilepsy, nerves, sexual disorders, tremors, vitality
Conception/ Central	CH	Holds past traumatic events	Releases pre-birth and birth trauma, and allows energy to circulate	Birth and pre-birth trauma, fatigue, indecision, panic, shame, trauma, worry	Abdomen, backache, chest, coldness, face, fibroids, hernia, lumps, lungs, menopause, nerves, reproductive problems, throat, weakness

Meridian	Point	When Blocked	When Tapped	Psychological	Physical
Kidney	CB	Low energy, poor decision-making	Helps willpower and impetus to carry out tasks	Gentleness, willpower, impetus to carry out tasks	Ageing, accident proneness, backache, balance problems, bones, chronic tiredness, congenital diseases, developmental irregularities, hereditary diseases, ears, endocrine imbalances, energy level for activity, exhaustion, genetic inheritance, hearing problems, hormonal imbalances, kidneys, osteoporosis, physical development, puberty, reproductive problems, sexual activity, stumbling, teeth, vertigo, weakness
Spleen	UA	Slows down thinking	Increases concentration and improved thinking patterns	Addictions, anxiety, decision-making	Anaemia, appetite, over-eating, bleeding disorders, diabetes, food digestion, digestive enzymes, hypoglycemia, periods, weight problems
Lung	TH	Lethargy and low energy	Releases negativity and increases positivity and vitality	Courage, disdain, intolerance, obsessive compulsive disorder, righteousness	Asthma, breathing disorders, tightness in chest, coughing, dry skin, eczema, emphysema, lungs, nasal congestion, nose, spots

Meridian	Point	When Blocked	When Tapped	Psychological	Physical
Large Intestine	IF	Nostalgia and harking for past	Releases emotions and causes us to live in the past. Increases goal-setting skills and optimism	Guilt, living in the past, wellbeing	Bowels, catarrh, constipation, diarrhoea, digestion, diverticulitis, irritable bowel syndrome, intestinal problems, mucus, nasal congestion, sinuses, skin
Circulation Sex	MF	Low self-esteem	Increases willpower and releases inferiority	Advancing, humour, jealousy, regret, sex problems, unhappiness, willpower	Hardening of arteries, angina, blood pressure, tightness of chest, circulation, heart disease, inhalant-type allergies, palpitations, sex problems, veins
Heart	LF	Chest pains, loneliness and selfishness	Develops empathy, compassion and unconditional love. Removes limited thinking	Compassion, consciousness, empathy, joy, unconditional love	Central nervous system, circulation, heart disease, night sweats, speech disorders, sweat glands, tongue
Small Intestine	KC	Lack of confidence, self-hate	Removes self-doubt, feelings of low self-esteem and improves confidence	Anxiety, cloudy judgement, lack of confidence, decision-making, doubt, self-hate, low self-esteem, mind clarity, shock, sadness, self-doubt, thinking processes	Abdominal pain, anaemia, circulation, gas, nutrient absorption, small intestine
Triple Warmer	GS	Inability to express love and emotions	Opens us to emotional interaction with others	Emotional coldness, communication, depression, low self-esteem, loneliness, living in the past, past problems, repressed emotions, resentment, self-hate, unsociability	Allergies, bladder, chilliness, fluid retention, heat regulation, immune system, infections (low resistance, intestinal problems) separation and evacuation, kidneys, liver, breathing, lymphatic system, physical pain, toxins, spleen, stomach

TROUBLESHOOTING

•••

My score will not go down

• •

Are you tapping for the right thing? A problem can often have many different faces. The technique WILL work if you are addressing the right thing. If a wheel has fallen off your car, and you change the exhaust, the car will still not go.

Sometimes these things take a little perseverance. Are you familiar with the children's game where you make a sandcastle and put a coin on the top? Each child takes turns in taking a scoop from the sand, and eventually the sand collapses into a pile. Your problem is the coin, and the scooping is done with EFT. The pile of sand is your emotions connected with the problem. If there is only one emotion (e.g. shame), then the problem will only need one scoop! However, as there are normally many aspects to each problem, you need to treat each of these individually before the coin will drop.

Are you tapping the right points? Check the positioning on the chart entitled **The Meridians, Points and How They Affect You** on pages 180-183. My website also has video clips of me tapping all the points correctly.

I have tried all of that and it is still not working

There are such things called 'energy toxins'. These prevent the technique from having its full effect. Unfortunately, they are difficult to trace, but fortunately rare. Try drinking water, changing rooms, changing clothes, sitting in a different chair, etc. The toxin may be in the fabric of the clothes you wear or something you have eaten. Go without tea/coffee three hours before a session and drink plenty of water.

You could also choose to do one of the breathing exercises explained in Unit 7. They will help the meridians to flow evenly and in the right direction.

If none of these work, then have a shower without using soaps of any kind and try again. If there is still no result, then the toxin has probably been ingested. Virtually anything can be toxic to your body and therefore interfere with your energy system. The most likely candidates are those things that you eat lots of. Try cutting these out for a couple of days and trying again. The most common items (though they may not

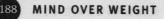

be toxic to you) are as follows: perfume, herbs, wheat, corn, refined sugar, coffee, tea, caffeine, alcohol, nicotine, dairy, pepper. Bear in mind that your intuition is often accurate. What do you think it is?

How do I tap?

Tapping should be done fairly firmly but not enough to bruise yourself! If a point hurts, instead of tapping just hold the point for two breaths. If you physically cannot tap a point, then don't worry, you could imagine tapping it or miss it out altogether. You should tap about seven times fairly quickly.

Are there any shortcuts?

After you have used the technique for a little while, you may find that you can omit The Setup stage and often The Gamut Procedure. This will leave you with The Sequence and The Sequence Repeated. If any points really 'do the trick' for you, i.e. they are really effective, then try using just these. The rule is to try it and see — you can always go back and do the complete technique.

USEFUL CONTACTS AND FURTHER INFORMATION

● ●

Websites

Try these websites for more information:

www.ilivelifefree.com — My own site with news, reviews, video clips of all of the tapping points, discussion board and details of courses and events.

www.emofree.com — Gary Craig's website. Packed with information and case histories.

HIGHLY RECOMMENDED

www.theamt.com — For Meridian Therapies in the UK

www.healthypages.co.uk — Good reference point for therapists and seekers

www.jbennette.com — A therapist in the US. Some useful information here.

www.meridian-therapy.com — Association for the Advancement of Meridian Therapies, listings of practitioners and training events.

www.energytherapies.org — Chrissie Hardisty is a Director of the AMT. This site is a good reference point.

http://members.aol/TickhillHealth — Dr Tam Llewellyn-Edwards Phd has a clinic in South Yorkshire where he works alongside therapists of other disciplines

Private Treatment

To find an EFT practitioner in your area you may email me at **referral@ilivelifefree.com** with your contact details, and I will put you in touch. Alternatively, you may telephone free on 0800 083 0796 during normal office hours. This is normally an answer phone service.

COURSES FROM LIVELIFEFREE

• •

UNDERSTANDING YOUR WEIGHT – A JOURNEY INTO THE UNCONSCIOUS

COURSE OBJECTIVE

'Understanding your Weight' is a weekend course that is designed to be fun, factual and effective. The purpose of the weekend is to help delegates understand their unconscious minds and the role that it plays in their weight. We aim to help you uncover, and eliminate, all those blocks and barriers that prevent weight loss.

COURSE AIMS

1. The delegate will be able to identify emotional causes that affect their weight.
2. The delegate will learn a new technique, namely EFT™ that will enable the individual to eliminate those causes.
3. The delegate will be able to understand the role that the unconscious mind has on their weight.
4. The delegate will be supported in an atmosphere of confidence, trust and compassion.

OTHER PUBLICATIONS BY THE AUTHOR

● ●

I Will Pass My Driving Test

Published by John Blake publishing, *I Will Pass My Driving Test* offers a host of practical tips on how to pass your test and explores the blocks that prevent many people from passing.

ISBN 1 904034 02 0